LIVING WITH A
HEARING LOSS

6| 2175157

This book is dedicated
to my wife Diana, whose
encouragement and support
have been a continual
inspiration to me.

Living with a hearing loss

Kenneth Edwards

A. & A. Farmar

British Library Cataloguing in Publication Data
A CIP catalogue record for this book is available
from the British Library
ISBN 978-1-906353-14-8

First published in 2009
by
A. & A. Farmar Ltd
78 Ranelagh Village, Dublin 6, Ireland
Tel +353-1-496 3625 e-mail afarmar@iol.ie
website www.aafarmar.ie
Printed and bound by GraphyCems

Contents

The tale of Alfie Grey

This is the tale of Alfie Grey
whose hearing had almost passed away.
Said Alfie, who was never afraid,
'I'll buy myself a hearing aid.'

It was no sooner said than done —
he had a test and then tried one.
'This is great,' he said at last,
'I can hear just as well as I did in the past.'

But going into the street once more
he couldn't hear for the traffic roar.
'I can't hear anything now,' he said
and was so depressed he went to bed.

'That was a total waste of cash —
I wish I'd never had a bash.'
His wife came in with a cup of tea
and the latest **Hearsay** *for him to see.*

'What's this,' he said, 'a lip-reading class?
Now that is something I just can't pass.'

Going along he quickly found
his wasn't the only problem around.

He wasn't the only one at all
so many others had had their fall.
The classes were a great success
although he really had to confess

'At reading lips I'm not much good
but I've learnt a lot, just as I should,
about other things apart from lips
which is great for those whose hearing slips.

A hearing aid can be a gift—
learn its use and it will give you a lift.
You don't just put it in and hear,
—you must learn to use it in your ear.'

So if you buy an aid today
give it a chance and don't throw it away.
Though it may not be quite what you thought
a wonderful friend is what you've bought.

*Before I started to lose my hearing, I
used to know Spring was here
when I could hear the birds
getting excited and chirping away.
I can't hear them any more, but now
I watch the daffodils dancing instead.
There is always something else
to appreciate, another way
to enjoy life.*

1 What's the big deal?

It's strange, isn't it, but people just do not seem to understand what it is like to have a hearing loss. After all, why should they? You look perfectly normal. You are not going around on crutches or with a white stick. They wonder why you are making such a fuss 'just because you can't hear very well'.

They never seem to catch on to the fact that it is not just lack of hearing that is the problem, but also the isolation that comes with it. Going out for the evening to the pub or to a film is no fun if you don't know what is going on. Not only is it no fun, it is also very frustrating. Your whole sense of communication has been destroyed or impaired.

When I started to lose my hearing, about forty years ago, I was devastated. My whole world seemed to collapse around my ears. Nothing was the same and everything was wrong. I could not hear the alarm in the morning. Speech was difficult to hear and on the telephone, it was almost impossible. One of my real loves was music—I used to sing in the RTÉ choral society. Suddenly that was gone and I could not even hear music properly. Going out to pubs or the theatre or even the films was an endurance test. I ran my own business and that also became so difficult that I wondered just how long I would be able to carry on and make a living. How could I earn money if I could not hear what people were saying to me? Suddenly everything seemed to be falling apart.

I could, and did, make a list of all the things I could not enjoy any more. The list grew longer and longer and everything seemed wrong and impossible. More and more I was feeling sorry for myself. Nobody seemed to understand.

I took time off and shut up business for a week. I went out walking to pass the time. One day, I was walking down the West Pier in Dún Laoghaire and when I got to the end of the pier I stopped to watch the fishermen casting their lines off the end of the pier. It was then that I noticed him. He was in a wheelchair and had no legs. He was chatting away to the others, baiting his hooks and casting out and thoroughly enjoying himself. I wondered to myself 'What has he got to be so happy about, sitting in a wheelchair with no legs?'

Then it hit me. He was doing what he could and enjoying it even though he had this terrible handicap. Here was I, perfectly normal except for my hearing, and nothing seemed right and I was thoroughly miserable. I felt ashamed of myself.

I walked back down the pier in full thought. When I got home I threw out all the lists I had made of the things I could not do any more. This time, I started a list of the things I could do. As the list grew and grew I began to realise just how fortunate I was in fact. It was the beginning of accepting my hearing loss and of putting it into perspective. For the first time it came to me that the only thing wrong with me was that I could not hear

Three useful rules

There are three simple rules that are worth following if you have hearing loss. They seem to help most people. I am not saying that they are easy to follow but they do work if you will let them. Do not forget that you have to work at having a hearing loss.

1. Accept that you have a hearing loss and make the best of it. Worrying will not change anything and can in fact make life more difficult. A sense of humour is a tremendous asset.

2. Don't try to hide the loss, you won't gain anything by it. Realise that other people have noticed your loss so it is best to be open about it and tell people. Keeping it to yourself only prevents others from being able to help you.

3. Tell other people what you find helpful. When people know what is best for you, they can be most helpful and this can remove a great deal of unnecessary strain on your part and on their part as well.

very well. Everything else was the same.

One of the first problems I had to deal with was the telephone. I had to use it in order to work and earn a living but I just could not hear on the one I had. I went along to the telephone people and asked them if there was a telephone with an amplification switch on it. As it so happened, there were few in those days, but they were available and after a little rooting around they found an old one. It was the last model they had. When I got it home I plugged it in and had a go, dialling the weather. The amplification was a great help and it seemed as if I just might be able to manage. Then I made a sudden discovery. I shifted the ear piece of the telephone up a little so that it was on my hearing aid and not on my ear. Suddenly I could hear, not perfectly, but it was much better. I had been using the old telephone in the wrong way. All at once life seemed so much brighter.

The next experiment was with the alarm clock. With my aid out, I could not hear the alarm going off. Special flashing and vibrating clocks are now available but I knew nothing about them then. I made do by putting the alarm clock in an open biscuit tin. That concentrated the sound and I was just able to hear it. Things were looking up.

What I was learning was that there were new ways of looking at and doing things. Many of the things I had just taken for granted had to be rethought. I was learning to accept my hearing loss and to make changes to my lifestyle so that I could cope and also continue to live and work happily. This may sound all about me, but it does illustrate a point. Once we accept that having a hearing loss is our lot, then we can make changes and still enjoy life to the full.

Like you, I have been through the mill and have had to face many of the difficulties you have to face. Because of this, I have decided to put down on paper my experiences of some of the things that have to be overcome or endured, and some of the ways we can help ourselves. Sharing difficulties can help us to accept them. It does not make the difficulties you face any easier to deal with but at least you

In the pub
Is going to the pub difficult because of the background noise? Some pubs have tiled or wooden floors that reflect every sound. Pubs with hard floors generate extra noise as well as reflecting the sound around and making it worse. But it may be possible to find a pub with a thick carpet and heavy curtains that help to absorb some of the background noise.

know that you are not the only one and are not on your own. Seeing how others cope with the same kinds of problems that you are confronted with influences you and helps you to cope in a better way.

Things are not as bleak and lonely as they were forty years ago, mind you, because there was very little help available in those days. There was nobody I could go to for advice, or if there was, I did not know about them. Nowadays, there are associations and groups that understand and can help you to cope. Legislation has improved somewhat as well so that help is available to some, if not all, who suffer. Having said all that, a hearing loss can be a very lonely, depressing and frustrating disability to have—and it is a disability, make no mistake about it.

Many people fight their loss and pretend nothing is wrong at all. They will not accept that they have dificulty hearing and persuade themselves that if only other people would talk clearly, they would have no problem at all. I did this myself when I first started to lose my hearing. I blamed everyone else.

I used to say 'If everyone spoke properly I would be able to hear perfectly well.' It was so easy to blame others and, of course, that meant I did not have to do anything myself. It was not until I misinterpreted something one day and one of my children told me that I should have my ears washed out, that I suddenly realised other people saw that I was having difficulties. It made me stop and think. It was only then that I admitted to myself that I could have a hearing loss of some kind.

The most difficult thing is to recognise that you have a problem and after that the next most difficult thing is admitting it to others. Some people just give up. To them, losing their hearing is the end. They give up going out because they are not able to hear and they just hibernate.

The main thing to remember is that once you accept your loss, it is possible to do something about it. The mistake I made was to concentrate on the things I could not do. If you zone in on the things you can do, then you are well along the way of acceptance. It is a good idea to make a little list. Think of the things you like and want to do and try to forget your loss for the moment.

Always remember one very important thing. The only thing wrong with you is that you cannot hear properly. Think

Pass the salt
The family were sitting around the kitchen table having a meal of corned beef. My mother turned to my uncle and said 'Pass the salt' and he said 'No, thank you.' We all looked at one another and burst out laughing. My uncle looked up and said 'No, I don't want parsley sauce, thank you.' When we told him what he had got wrong, he laughed as much as the rest of us.

about that for a moment. You are still the same person you were before your hearing started to go. You still have the same likes and dislikes as you had before. You still have the same capabilities and abilities. Nothing has changed except that your hearing has diminished.

Don't give up on life and stop going out just because you cannot hear. Find other ways to enjoy things or even new things to enjoy. The choice is yours. Do you give up or do you accept your new loss as a challenge and get out and do something about it?

Remember this. I was in the same boat and I have found that my hearing loss has given me so much. It may have taken much joy away from me, but it also opened up many doors and made me re-think everything I had previously done. It introduced me to many new ideas and new friends.

It is an extraordinary thing, but normally we tend to develop our own little habits and ways of doing things and get into a form of rut. It is only when there is an outside influence, like a bus strike, for example, that we have to do something different. We must walk to where we want to go, or get a lift, or get a train where in the past we went by bus. We can no longer do the things we used to do in the same way but we find a way around the difficulty. A hearing loss is a bit like this. Sometimes it is just a matter of trying a little harder to find an alternative or something else that is suitable for us. It is not a matter of giving up, it is a matter of making a change, possibly taking a new direction.

There are many ways of helping ourselves and we do not have to just give up. I would not wish a hearing loss on anyone, but if that is your lot, it is far better to accept it and turn it to your advantage than to sit and moan about how it has ruined your life. Get up and go out and enjoy yourself and do not give up: after all, you only have a hearing loss. Do not be afraid of making a mistake and you will find that most people do their best to help you if you will only let them. We all make silly mistakes and if we can learn to laugh at them, others will laugh with us.

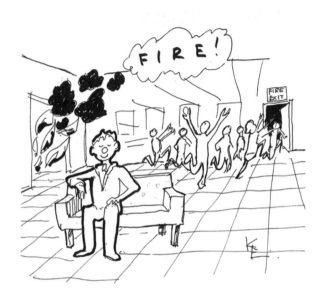

2 First steps

Losing your hearing is usually a very gradual process. Normally it does not happen overnight. I know that that can happen as well, but it is not all that frequent. For the majority of people with hearing loss, there is a gradual diminishing of the sound they can hear. It creeps up on them slowly. In addition, of course, most people just do not want to admit to having a loss. So realising that you have a hearing loss is not always easy.

Causes of hearing loss

Possibly the most common cause of hearing loss is old age, and this is the reason many people will not admit to having a loss in the first place. To do so admits to being old and few people want to do that.

Another cause is damage to the ear because of exposure to excessive loud sounds. There are two main kinds of loss associated with exposure to very loud sounds. The first one is a temporary diminishing of hearing after being exposed to loud noise. This is known as 'temporary threshold shift'. Normally the hearing will return after a short while. An explosion or a very loud sudden noise can damage the ears permanently but this usually occurs only in the ear that was closest to the loud noise.

The second kind of loss is permanent and is caused by exposure to long periods of loud noise, for example at work. The hearing can gradually deteriorate and this normally takes place in both ears. This is why it is so important to protect your ears if you work in very noisy places.

Working in a very noisy environment is not the only cause of hearing loss. Even frequent visits to discos, where the noise level can be horrendous, can be damaging to the ears. It is noticeable that more and more young people are acquiring a hearing loss and this can be caused by the excessive sound level in places of entertainment.

Unfortunately there's no treatment
Remember that there is no treatment that can revive the hearing once the ear has been damaged. Prevention is the only hope for those who are exposed to continual loud sound, in their workplace, for example, and this is by means of ear protectors.

Sometimes hearing loss may be caused by some medical problem which can be rectified. Sometimes it can be due to wax in the ear. When the wax is removed, the hearing may be restored. With children, glue ear may also be a problem.

Tinnitus

Even worse than having a hearing loss is to have tinnitus as well. It can add greatly to the problems of being hard of hearing. Occasionally tinnitus occurs without any hearing loss due to an infection or other event.

Continual sounds are heard which arise from the hearing mechanism itself. These are usually described as continual hissing, ringing, buzzing or knocking noises. They just won't go away. The sound is always there. At the moment there is no cure for tinnitus. Once the hair cells to the inner-ear are damaged, they cannot be restored. The only thing to be done is to learn to cope with the noise. It will not go away.

Tinnitus seems worse under very quiet circumstances, for example at night when trying to sleep. It can help to try to mask the sound by introducing another one. One way of doing this is by means of a tinnitus masker. This is a little like a hearing aid which gives out a soft, gentle sound. The ear tends to hear that sound and not the sound from the tinnitus.

Go to your GP first

If you feel your hearing is not as good as it should be, the first thing to do is to go to your GP—do not go out and buy a hearing aid without seing your doctor first. A friend of mine told me that he went to a hearing aid supplier first because he thought his hearing had got worse. He was lucky, the supplier was an honest man and would not sell him an aid—he told him that he had wax in his ears and should go to see his GP. When the wax was cleaned out, my friend could hear perfectly again. He could easily have been sold an expensive aid, or even two, by an unscrupulous supplier.

So, go to your GP first and let him or her have a look. If all you need is to have your ears washed out then you are lucky. But if your GP suspects you have a permanent hearing loss the next step is to have your hearing tested.

If you have a medical card your GP can refer you to the Health Services Executive (HSE). They will put you in touch with your local board's audiology service for a hearing test. Do not be put off by people saying that it will take twelve months to hear from them. I went myself and was seen within two months. A lot depends on what district you are in; some are quicker than others depending on circumstances.

The audiologist will evaluate your hearing loss and may recommend an aid which will be supplied by the HSE.

If you do not have a medical card your GP may send you to an ENT (ear, nose and throat) specialist. The specialist can test your hearing and establish if indeed you have got a hearing loss and can recommend what will suit you best. The specialist may also recommend a hearing aid supplier but if you do need an aid you don't necessarily have to go to the supplier the specialist suggests—the choice is up to you. But do be careful. There are many hearing aid suppliers around and many are excellent but some are not as good as they should be. (See Chapter 3 on how to choose an audiologist and/or aid supplier.)

If you go to an ENT consultant, do plan your visit before you go and do not do what I did. Many years ago I went for a hearing test with an ENT consultant in Dublin. Of course, I was very apprehensive before I went. When I arrived at the black and forbidding hall door, I rang the bell. There must have been a click or a buzz or something but I heard nothing. Eventually I pushed the door and it opened and I went into a dull and dreary hall. A small sign pointed to 'Reception' and I duly followed. When I got there, I said I had an appointment. The receptionist was looking down at her books and mumbled something. I could not hear her. 'What?' I said. She repeated something but I still did not hear her.

When I had eventually heard what she wanted and answered her questions and she had finished interrogating me, she sent me into the waiting room. There were three or four people scattered around looking unhappy. I took a seat opposite the door. After twenty minutes or so, the receptionist came in, shouted something and disappeared again. Nobody moved. Had I missed something again? She came back after a while and came over to me and told me I could go to see the specialist now.

It was all exasperating and it was then that I realised how badly I had managed the whole thing. To start with, I should have brought someone with me who had good hearing. They could have filled in all the bits that I had missed. This is particularly important for your first visit when you have no hearing aid to help you. Failing that, I should have organised my mind better. If I had gone in and said my name, the time of my appointment and the name of the specialist, the receptionist could have thought of very little to ask me. I could also have told her that I would not hear her when she announced my name in the waiting room and that she would have to come over to me. These little things would have made such a difference.

Do think about what you are going to say before you go, it is well worth while. In my case, it would also have been better if the receptionist had faced me and spoken to me instead of to her books. I might well have heard her a little better. This lack of understanding from the receptionist of an ENT specialist is unacceptable.

Personally, I have not found many ENT specialists much better than this

Let's have a drink
Three elderly men were sitting in the park on a very blustery day. They were all rather hard of hearing.
'Windy, isn't it?' one of them said.
'Not at all,' the second one said, 'it's Thursday.'
'I'm thirsty too,' the third man said.

receptionist at talking to people with a hearing impairment. ENT consultants are highly qualified people but that does not mean that they understand what it is like to have a hearing loss. I have been to several specialists now and although they have been able to discover exactly what was wrong with me, they did not seem to realise the trauma and apprehension that sufferers go through. I was simply told that I had a hearing loss and that I should go to an audiologist and have a hearing aid fitted. 'It might help,' I was told.

To me this was devastating and I well remember thinking that the specialist was just handing me over to someone else because he could do nothing for me. He did not even seem to know if it would help or not. 'It might help,' he had said. I felt abandoned. I know perfectly well that this was probably sound advice and that I did need a hearing aid, but the suddenness and lack of sensitivity with which the diagnosis was given made me realise how unaware the specialist was of my apprehensions and fears.

This may seem very critical but it is not

6| 2175157

based on my own experiences alone. I have had letters from many people who have had similar experiences. I have also talked to people who had tinnitus and an ENT consultant had told them that hearing aids would not help them in the least. Eventually, they went to audiologists who fitted aids and they found them very helpful. I do realise that hearing aids may not be suitable or helpful for some tinnitus sufferers, but that is not necessarily true for all. If there is any chance that an aid might be helpful the patient should be told—it seems to me almost criminal to advise against an aid when it might help someone lead a reasonably normal life.

I am not knocking ENT consultants generally and I know there are many who are excellent at communicating, but I do wish that some of them would be more tuned in to the psychological problems and apprehensions of patients with a hearing loss. This is where a hearing companion is helpful as they can hear exactly what is being said and recommended.

In the next chapter, I will give you some advice on how to choose a qualified, competent audiologist who will recommend the best type of hearing aid for you and will not try to sell you an aid simply for the money.

Mr Jones isn't well

'I saw Mr Jones today and he doesn't look well at all.'

'Does he not, poor man?'

'He looks wretched. He's got angina.'

'That's silly then, going to China when he's not well.'

'He's not going to China.'

'You just said he was.'

'No, I didn't. I said he had angina.'

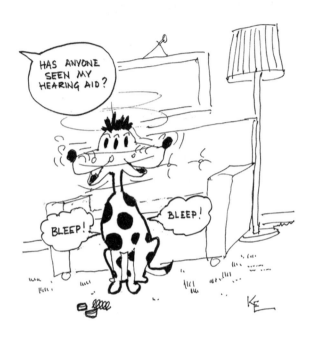

3. Getting your hearing tested

It is extremely important if you go to have your ears tested by an audiologist in private practice that you choose one who is properly qualified and is not just trying to sell you an aid. Most audiologists supply aids, as well as evaluating patients' hearing, and they may try to sell you these

A sense of humour
The first time I went to an audiologist to get an aid, he tested my ears and eventually fitted me with an aid and mould. I asked him how much all this was going to cost me? When he told me the price I said 'What?' He told me once more and I innocently said 'What?' again. He than realised he was being had and he smiled and I well remember what he said to me. He said 'A sense of humour will help you a lot.' He was so right

aids even if they are not the most suitable.

There are also certain dangers in being treated by unqualified audiologists. They may diagnose problems incorrectly. They may also miss or be unaware of a serious problem that needs medical attention. Even supplying a hearing aid with an incorrect pitch can cause additional damage to the hearing.

Qualified audiologists are trained to spot other things apart from the degree of hearing loss and in certain cases can refer patients to an ENT specialist for treatment.

The European Communities (Medical Devices) Regulation 1994 regulates the prescription and fitting of hearing aids but this regulation is not enforced in Ireland. Most European countries have a register of professional audiologists but this is not the case in Ireland. However, all the members of the Irish Society of Hearing Aid Audiologists are qualified and accredited so you should have no problems if you go to one of their members. They have the letters MISHAA or FISHAA after their name. The Society's register of members is available on their website www.ishaa.ie

According to the Society, a significant number of those fitting hearing aids in Ireland have no relevant professional qualifications. They may have letters after

When choosing a hearing aid supplier

- Check that the audiologist is fully qualified and accredited with the Irish Society of Hearing Aid Audiologists.
- Choose an audiologist whose premises are easily accessible.
- Check whether you are eligible for a grant or grants under the Treatment Benefit Scheme.
- If you are eligible for a grant check that the supplier you have chosen is registered with the Department of Social and Family Affairs.
- Check that you can return the aid if it is not satisfactory and get your money back.
- Check that the audiologist is available to service your aid if it breaks down.

A free hearing aid?
The only really free hearing aids are those supplied and fitted on a medical card. Those aids are very good but at the moment include only the older analogue types. The digital types are not yet supplied to medical card holders.

their names but these may simply refer to an Internet course.

If you live in a city or large town be sure to go to someone who has a proper office, and not a hotel room. However, in smaller places there may not be enough demand for a permanent establishment and some excellent and well-established audiologists take hotel rooms there. Some will also go to a private house if the person is bed-ridden. But do be careful and ask and find out as much as possible.

When you have satisfied yourself that the audiologist you are thinking of going to is qualified and is available to service your aid if it breaks down, see if any of your friends also attended that audiologist and if so whether they were satisfied with the service they got. Then make your choice.

Beware of going to an audiologist who advertises free aids, or comes to your house to test you, unless you are bedridden. Do be cautious about adverts for free or cheap hearing aids. These are sometimes intended as a means of getting you along in the first place. In many instances, the free aids may be deemed unsuitable for you and the audiologist may well then try to sell you an expensive aid.

There have been many complaints about unqualified audiologists but the situation is tending to improve. The main point is that you should go to a supplier who has an established set-up and has a proper shop front and is in a position to give adequate support at a later stage and carry out repairs where necessary. It is no use having a hearing aid that cannot be repaired if it goes wrong. If you buy an aid from someone in a hotel room you may never see them again and if there is a problem later, you are on your own.

Grants for hearing aids

If you obtain a hearing aid privately, whether or not you hold a medical card, you may be eligible for a grant towards the cost of one, or even two, aids from the Department of Family and Social Affairs.

The Department operates the Treatment Benefit Scheme open to patients with full PRSI cover and who fulfill other eligibility criteria. At the time of writing the grant covered 50 per cent of the cost up to €830 of a hearing aid, and was available with or without a medical card. Be careful, though, because grants are not available to everyone; eligibility seems to depend on your taxation bracket so it is wise to check on www.welfare.ie if you are eligible before you commit yourself to buying. You just may not get the grant.

Ear tests

Once you have decided on a hearing aid supplier who fulfils all these requirements, the next step is to have your ears fully tested.The test covers four main areas: case history, otoscopy, tympanometry and audiometry. Let us take each of these separately and very simply.

The case history is almost self explanatory and involves noting down all your personal details. These include questions about your hearing, exposure to noise at work and elsewhere, whether you wear a hearing aid and whether you suffer from dizziness, tinnitus and so on. These questions are all important in helping the consultant or audiologist to understand your problems. Once again, a hearing companion can be of great help in communicating what is being said to you.

Otoscopy involves an examination of each ear using a form of illuminating magnifying glass called an otoscope. This allows an examination of the ear canal and can show up wax or blockages or any other problems. (One of the consultants I went to was talking to me as he did this. I could not see him because he was out of my line of vision and he had the otoscope stuck in my ear. I do not quite know how he expected me to hear him.)

Tympanometry is a method of testing the ear to see how it moves in response to pressure. A small probe is inserted into the ear cavity and the patient may hear some loud bleeps. The test is meant to establish if anything is inhibiting the motion of the eardrum, such as an infection or fluid.

An audiometric test is carried out in a soundproof room. The patient is equipped with a pair of ear phones and is required to indicate when certain sounds or tones which come through the ear phones are heard. This is done by raising the hand each time a sound is heard or by pressing a buzzer. Air conduction is tested by this means when soft tones are used. Bone conduction is tested by placing a bone vibrator behind the ear, bypassing the outer and middle ear altogether, and only stimulated by means of the inner ear directly.

Types of hearing loss

These ear tests help to establish what kind of hearing loss there is. It may be conductive, which is a loss in the outer ear. It may be sensorineural where the loss is in the inner ear or it may be mixed and is both conductive and sensorineural. An audiogram is used to record the threshold of each pitch for each ear. This record of the examination can, of course, be stored and used to establish any improvement or depreciation in the hearing at a future date.

When the type of hearing loss you have has been established the next step is to choose a hearing aid or aids. Do remember that while the audiologist may suggest a particular type of aid you are the expert. Only you know what you can hear and it is sometimes helpful to try out different types of aid to see which helps you most.

There are very many different types of hearing aids available to you. Take a look at the next chapter to see what I mean.

.

4. Choosing and learning to use your hearing aid

There are so many types and makes of hearing aid available it can be very confusing trying to choose between them. Some will be suitable for you while others may not help with the kind of hearing loss you have.

Usually the make or brand is dictated by the supplier you go to for your test, although some offer aids from a wide range of manufacturers. Most of the makes seem to be good and reliable. Personally, I would not be too concerned about the manufacturer of the aid. It is more important that the supplier is qualified and can give good backup. Another important factor is how easy it is to get to the supplier. Try to choose one who is nearby or readily accessible. If something goes wrong, it is very helpful if you can get to your supplier quickly and easily.

The digital aids now available are a great improvement on the old analogue type aid (which is still the only type available on the medical card). They are fitted with tiny computers which can assess the type of sound being received and automatically adjust the volume accordingly. That is the theory, at any rate. The aids can be personalised and can be tuned to your type of hearing by the audiologist. This can certainly be an advantage.

Early models had no manual volume control and when I tested one, I found it impossible to hear under some circumstances. In theory, the aid should have adjusted itself automatically according to the level of sound. In practice, I found it terrible. I had no control over it at all and when it turned down automatically I could hear very little. I gave it back after a week.

I did not get another digital aid until they had manual volume control and I found this was essential for me. What suits my kind of hearing does not necessarily suit yours. It is your hearing and only you will know if the aid suggested will be suitable for you.

There are also directional aids. These have two small microphones installed. The aid can pick up sounds coming from the front (the direction of most speech) far better than sounds coming from the side or from behind. With some aids it is possible to switch to the appropriate microphone in the aid depending on the kind of noise situation you happen to be in. This sounds far more complicated than it is and it can be helpful for some people. I tried an aid of this kind at one time but found that I became far more aware of my hearing loss and was switching away for the appropriate sound all the time. In the end, I gave up and gave the aid back again. It just did not work for me. It might help you, though.

Behind-the-ear aids

The workhorse of the hearing aid range is the behind-the-ear type. It rests behind the ear and has a plastic tube connection to an ear mould set into the ear. This is by far the most common type and is comfortable to wear and easy to use. Although the mould itself can be seen in the ear, the aid behind the ear is usually hidden by the hair. Some manufacturers, for example the Swiss firm PHLOX, make aids with the housing coloured to blend in with the colour of the hair.

These aids have simple controls and because of their reasonable size it is easy

The very small aids

Most people do not want to advertise the fact that they have a hearing loss and want one of those tiny aids that go in the ear and are nearly invisible. However, these may not be suitable for the kind of loss you have.

Obviously the smaller the aid, the less power can be crammed into it. If your hearing is very poor, an in-the-ear aid may not be powerful enough.

You are doing yourself no favours if you go for the vanity of not having it seen over the practicality of having a more conspicuous larger one with which you can hear properly.

to use the various controls. They come in various sizes and they can be suitable even for people who suffer from an extremely severe loss. There is an on/off switch or mechanism, a battery container and a volume control. Normally, but not always, they have what is called a T-switch which you will need in order to use some telephones and loop systems. (See page 128 for an explanation.) It is most important to choose an aid that does have a T-switch. You may not think you will use it, but you will find you want it if it isn't there.

Maintenance is low for these aids and on the whole they are very reliable. The plastic tubing will have to be renewed from time to time because the tube can

A small pad of cotton wool
Sometimes after prolonged use of a behind-the-ear aid, the top of the ear can become a little sore where the tube rubs it. I find that a small pad of cotton wool, which is invisible under the hair, can act as a temporary pad until the soreness goes. A little Savlon or cream will help a lot as well.

go hard after some time and the joints between tube and mould, and between tube and aid, can leak and give out a kind of whistling sound called 'feedback'.

Canal hearing aids

Another kind of aid is the canal hearing aid. This is very small and in fact seems to get smaller all the time. It is still visible in the ear but is less so than the mould of the behind-the-ear type. This is for the person who wants to hear better without the aid being too obvious. If your hearing loss is severe, this is probably not for you. With this kind of aid, the ear mould and the works are all in one. Everything is installed into this tiny ear-shaped shell.

Because of the small size of the aid, the controls are tiny and sometimes fiddly to use. These aids are less reliable than the behind-the-ear type and break down more. Because of their tiny size, they do not always have a T-switch.

These aids can be a little difficult to take out and are sometimes provided with a tiny piece of plastic so that you can get a grip on them. They are so comfortable to wear it is quite possible to forget you have an aid in at all. Beware when you take a shower or bath—you might well still be wearing your aid and have forgotten to take it out. It is easier than you think.

All-in-the-ear aid

The all-in-the-ear aid is very similar to the canal aid but is a little larger and can be more powerful as well. It is also far more visible; it can be seen from the side and it fills the main cavity of the ear. Being larger, the controls are easier to manipulate and less fussy. Once again, not all are fitted with T switches.

Completely-in-the-canal aid

There is now an even tinier aid available known as the completely-in-the-canal aid. This is almost totally invisible but is only of use to people who have a mild or slight hearing loss.

Spectacle hearing aids

Spectacle hearing aids are now available which have the aids set into the ends of the ear pieces. These can be for either bone or air conduction. The spectacle aid can be fitted to modern frames of your choice. These seem to be very efficient but remember, if you take your glasses off you will not be able to hear a thing. You need to wear your glasses all the time.

Ear moulds

If you are going to have an in-the-ear or a behind-the-ear aid the audiologist will take an impression of the inside of your ear. It is absolutely essential that the mould fits perfectly in your ear otherwise air can get past it and cause whistling or feedback. A form of pliable plasticine is packed carefully into your ear and

Picking the right glasses
If you wear glasses all the time you can find that the space behind the ear becomes overfilled with aid and tube as well as the ear pieces of the glasses. When choosing new frames be sure to wear your aid while trying the new glasses. Pick something with very narrow ear pieces and never mind the fashions. Too much behind the ears can make them very tender and sore.

allowed to set and then very carefully removed. This gives a perfect impression of the shape of the ear. It will then be sent away so that a mould can be made.

The mould can be in hard or soft plastic. It is a matter of taste but the soft type is supposed to be better. I have two aids, and I have a soft mould in one and a hard one in the other. I don't know why, but they suit me at the moment.

There will be a wait of about a week or so while your ear mould is being made especially for you. You will then have to go back and have your aid properly fitted and tuned. The mould should fit perfectly and snugly and it should not hurt. If you feel any pain or discomfort tell the audiologist immediately. Sometimes the slightest sanding of a part of the mould will make an enormous difference. Do not go away with a pain in your ear.

Cost of hearing aids

Another important aspect of getting your aid, if it is not being supplied on a medical card, is cost. Aids are very expensive and there can be hidden costs if you are not careful. Find out if the price quoted allows for hearing tests and fitting. Also, be sure what the guarantee is. After the guarantee period, which is normally about two years, you will be responsible for paying for any repairs. Your supplier should be in a position to carry out these repairs or have them done quickly.

You may be eligible for a grant towards the cost of your aid or aids: see page 30 for details.

One or two hearing aids?

Are there any advantages in having two hearing aids? Many audiologists now recommend two and of course, this doubles the amount of money you are being asked to pay out. Personally, I use two aids. I have about 85 per cent loss in my left ear and my right ear is almost useless.

When I applied for two new aids on my medical card, my ears were tested and the audiologist felt that it was useless giving me a second aid for my right ear. I explained that sometimes by accident I would forget that I had not switched on my right aid and after a while I became aware that I was missing a great deal of conversation.

When checking both aids and discovering that the right aid was turned off, I switched it on and found that I could hear much better. This may sound odd, because although I can hear no real speech from the right ear, even with the aid switched on, it does help me to hear

You are the expert
Specialists may test your ears and tell you precisely how much loss you have but in fact, only you know what you can hear. You do have to try aids in your own surroundings to be sure that they are suitable for you. It does not matter in the least if the specialist says that a certain aid is most suitable for you. He or she may well be right, and it can get you started on a particular model. At the same time, it is not until you are happy with the results yourself that you can be sure that the aid you are getting works for you. Nobody can tell you what you can hear. Only you know that.

with the other ear. It seems to give a better, more rounded sound and it is certainly an improvement for me to have two aids. I am not saying that this would be the case for everyone, but it works for me.

I got my two free aids in the end. Other people I know cannot manage using two aids. They have tried them and it just doesn't work for them. The main thing is not to be bullied or rushed into buying two aids. Try one first and see what the results are like. It is always possible to go back at some later stage and invest in the second aid, but do take your time. If you have reasonable hearing in both ears, two aids can help to improve the reduction of background noise.

Cochlea implants

Thee are much talked about these days. They are not for the hard of hearing though, only for those who are deaf and your hearing must be almost negligible so do not worry about this. The operation is carried out in the Beaumont Hospital in Dublin. Most people who have had this operation report that their hearing has improved.

Tuning and trying out your aid

Once your hearing aid has been fitted it has to be tuned to your own personal requirements, particularly if it is a digital aid. Of course, this will be done in a comfortable soundproof room but things will be quite different when you get out into the world where you live and it will take some time to adjust.

You have to find out what is best for you. This is why you are the expert. It is so important that you insist on a trial period for testing your new aid with a money-back guarantee. This means that if your new aid is not to your satisfaction you can do something about it and you are not stuck. Go to someone else if the audiologist is not prepared to give you that guarantee.

If you are having problems after a few days, go back again to your supplier and ask if adjustments can be made so that the aid meets your needs better. Do not forget that you are the expert. Nobody else has hearing just like you. Most audiologists have proper hearing and are greatly influenced by the claims of the hearing aid manufacturers. To really grasp just how good an aid is, it has to be worn in everyday conditions and only the hard of hearing person can do this.

Learning to use your aid

Having got a hearing aid, it is easy to imagine that you will be able to hear once again and everything will be all right. But you do not just put it in your ear and then hear. Things do not work like that at all. This is the stage where many people give up and newly acquired aids end up in dressing-table drawers. Your new aid will help you to hear but you do have to learn how to use it so that it can be of benefit to you.

To start with, the sound you get from your new aid will not be like the sound you have been used to in the past. Sound will come across as though from a cheap, tinny radio. Many sounds that you could hear before your hearing started to go will just disappear. Some people can no longer hear the birds singing. Others do not hear the clock ticking any more. All sorts of sounds have vanished. Other noises are amplified and can become horrendous.

Street noises from lorries and buses can be deafening. You have to learn how to hear once again. You have to learn to protect yourself from unwanted noise.

The problem with all hearing aids is that they amplify everything. But that does not mean that you will hear everything. The speech you really want to hear is made louder but so is the background noise and this can sometimes be louder than the speech. This is one of the most annoying parts of hearing amplification. Digital aids do help considerably but they do not eliminate the problem.

You may be told that certain aids cut down on background noise. Do not take that too literally. They may cut down on background noise but they do not eliminate it. You have to try aids out in the normal everyday circumstances under which you live to establish if they are suitable for you. Testing them in the audiologist's soundproof room is not sufficient.

One man I knew was told that two hearing aids would be beneficial to him. A hearing aid supplier came and fitted him with two aids and handed him a very large bill at the same time. He was not told how to use them and the concentration of sound and loud noises disturbed him so much that he removed both of them and handed them back and swore he would never have an aid again. He still has no aid after almost ten years and he has lost out badly over those years. This was totally irresponsible of the audiologist; it looks as if he was only interested in making a quick sale and had no concern for the user at all.

Do not expect your new aid to give you back what you have lost. Be prepared to work to make it advantageous to you. When you leave the audiologist wearing your new aid and go into the street, it is a good idea to switch it off. When I got my first aid I did not know this and in fact, I made a bad mistake. Perhaps I was a little over-anxious. I just could not wait to see what I had bought. The hearing aid specialist's premises was on the first floor, and on leaving with my new aid installed, I thought I would take a look at it. I went to the toilet and took the aid out and looked at where I switched it on and off and at the volume control and it seemed quite simple. I was able to get it back in my ear again quite well and then I proceeded to go out on to the street.

I was deafened. The traffic noise blasted at me and I was devastated. I wasn't

Ear candles

I was at a hotel for a weekend break and they had an ear-candle service, so I tried it out. I must say I found it most relaxing. I had been having a little difficulty with feedback, but after the session, it cleared up like magic. These are not ordinary candles but are special BIOSUN ear candles. Each ear is tackled separately. The person lies down on one side, one of these candles is placed in their ear and then lit and left. The flames creates a vibration in the air which generates a gentle type of massage effect on the ear drum. It is claimed that it is soothing and helpful for ear noise and stress. On completion, they cut open the hollow candles and show you what has been extracted from your ear. It makes you think. Do not try this out yourself! It should be carried out by an expert.

expecting that. In the end I had to switch the aid off but my immediate reaction was that I had just bought something that was not going to help me at all. When I got back home, I discovered what had happened. After taking out the aid to look at it, I had accidentally turned up the volume control to full blast when I put it back in my ear again. That was why all the street sounds were greatly magnified. I had learned my lesson.

The sudden rush of hard sound can be off-putting and disturbing. When you get your first aid, take it easy and take your time. You could even take the aid out until you get home again into reasonably quiet and familiar territory. Don't rush it. When you are relaxed and sitting quietly, put the aid back in and get familiar with the sound you get. Don't overdo it, just take it easy. Listen to some of the sounds you would normally hear around you and see how the newly amplified sounds compare with what you heard before. Talk to someone in the kitchen and at the same time turn on the tap and let it run into the sink. Notice how the noise of the tap can blot out what the person is saying.

Your aid is picking up the background noise and speech is blotted out.

Try not to have your aid turned up too high. This can distort the sound you hear and can also increase the background noise. It may sound strange but too strong an amplification can prevent you from hearing properly. After about half an hour, switch off the aid or take it out for a while. Gradually increase the amount of time you have the aid switched on. Bit by bit try other things. Go outside and see how the street noises affect you. Learn what your aid can do for you. It can be a wonderful friend or a terrible enemy, depending on how you use it. Very many people give up after a short while. They just don't seem to be able to cope with the extra loud noises and background sound. You do have to work at it but it is well worth the effort.

His new hearing aid

A man was boasting about the new hearing aid he had bought when he was abroad. 'It has just about everything,' he said. 'It completely cuts out background noise. It is so well fitted that there is no feedback noise and it has anti-condensation tubing fitted as standard. It is totally waterproof and you can wear it in the shower and it is dog proof and indestructible.'

'That sounds wonderful,' his companion said, 'and how much was it?'

'Ten past eight,' the boaster said looking at his watch.

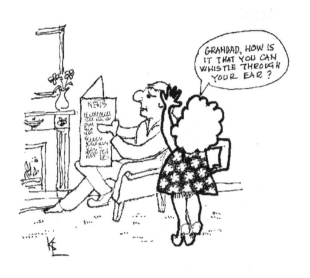

5 Looking after your aid

Your aid is a sensitive mechanism and should be treated with care. When you take it out, be careful where you put it. It is very light and can be swept away into some dark corner by a slight tap. Most important of all, it is essential to turn it off when you are not using it. This may sound obvious, but it is easy to forget.

If you leave it turned on, it will waste

Making life easier
There are many small items, such as magnatools (small screwdrivers with magnets), that can help to make life just a little easier for the hard of hearing. These small items are manufactured by Hal-Hen Company Inc. Some of the hearing aid suppliers may stock them or perhaps can get them for you.

your batteries, but more important, it can give off a continual high-pitched squeak or whistling sound. You will not be able to hear it because you are not wearing it. However, your pet may well hear it. A friend of mine left her aid on a low side table still switched on. Her pet dog got very interested and when she came back into the room, there was her dog in front of a small pile of little mechanical parts. It was her hearing aid.

It is essential not to let water near your aid. Once again be careful when having a shower. Have you forgotten to take your aid out? New aids and ear moulds can be so comfortable that it is quite possible to forget that you have them in at all. I was sitting in the bath once and suddenly remembered I still had my aid in. Fortunately, I was still sitting upright and I was able to take the aid out without damage. It was a near thing, though.

Condensation in the tube

If you are into strenuous exercise, for example, hill walking or something like that, you can get condensation in the little tube that joins the aid to the ear-mould. This is quite normal, but the little bubbles tend to block the tube and prevent sound from penetrating to your ear. It is necessary to remove the little bubbles. This can be done in several ways. My wife uses the simple method of taking out her aid and shaking it. This tends to unblock the tube.

Do be careful to hold it very firmly if you do it this way or your aid might fly out of your hand and end up somewhere it shouldn't be.

Another method that I use is to remove the aid and carefully pull the tube from the neck of the aid itself, not from the ear mould. You can then blow down the tube and remove all the bubbles quite simply. When you have done this, re-fix the tube to the aid and put it back in your ear. It is quite simple really. It is possible to get anti-condensation tubing fitted to your aid and this helps to reduce the condensation bubbles.

You could also get an earmould air blower to remove the condensation. It looks like a rubber or plastic bulb with a tiny nozzle and it can be used to remove moisture.

Excessive humidity can cause heavy perspiration and this can get into both tubes and even the hearing aid itself. There are Dri-Aid kits available that can help to remove damaging moisture. These are in the form of small plastic containers. All you have to do is place your aid and mould in the container and leave it overnight. You have to remove the batteries before doing this so do be careful where you put them.

Replacing the tubing

The tubing that joins the aid to the ear mould becomes hard with age. When this happens, the joints are not as tight as they should be and it can result in feedback, a kind of whistling. This tubing can be replaced very quickly by your supplier.

The tubing in the new digital aids needs to be replaced more frequently than the tubing in the old analogue aids. When you become more accustomed to your aid, you should be able to replace this tubing yourself, if you are handy at this kind of thing. It is quite simple. Next time you are with your supplier having it replaced, watch carefully to see how it is done.

Spare batteries

Be sure that you always carry some spare batteries around with you. You never know just when your battery will pack up so it is best to be sure.

Try to have a certain time each week when you replace the batteries. I do it every Saturday morning when I get up. This means that normally I don't get any unpleasant surprises when I am out or talking to someone important. Of course, this also means that the batteries you throw away are not quite dead, but I find this method best for me. You do what is best for you.

Replacing tiny batteries

Some modern hearing aids are really quite tiny and the batteries needed to run them are even tinier. They are so small that many people, especially more elderly people or those with some impaired vision, find it extremely difficult to extract the old used battery and replace it with a new one. It is difficult to get your fingers around it to extract it. A very useful tool to help with this is a small magnatool which is a little like a small screwdriver with a magnet attached to the end. With this, it is easy to extract the old battery and it can be used to put in the new one as well.

A word of advice, though. Do not change your battery on the bus or somewhere like that. Try to be at a table. If you drop your new battery it could go anywhere and never be found and it just might be the last one you have with you.

A roll and a beer
Going out the door I shouted 'I won't be long. I'm just going for a stroll down the pier.'
My wife called back, 'Don't drink too much.'
Perplexed, I came back in and asked, 'What do you mean?'
She said 'Don't drink too much when you have your roll and beer.'

6 Adapting to your new life

Over the years as a normal hearing person, you have built up many ways of doing things and do most of them without thinking. They have become almost automatic to you. For example, you might go into the local pub for a drink on the way home, just as a matter of course. Perhaps you sit over your dinner with the television on, watching the news or a favourite programme. Maybe you have your neighbour in for a cup of tea every Monday morning at eleven o'clock. There are so many things that have just become a habit. You do them without thinking, really.

When you lose your hearing, it is not always possible to enjoy these things in the same way. If you go to the pub, the background noise can be so great that you cannot hear a thing. Maybe it is a strain to hear the television and eat at the same time. Perhaps you cannot hear your friend with the washing machine going. There are still many ways of enjoying yourself, but not necessarily from the things you did in the past.

These are just a few examples, but not all of the habits you have built up will be as enjoyable as they were when your hearing was all right. It is not always possible to carry on as before but that does not mean that you give up. It simply means that, if you want to, you can still find things that give you pleasure and enjoyment. This can only be done if you are prepared to make changes in your lifestyle.

Douglas Bader, the war-time fighter pilot, who lost both his legs, had been a great sportsman. When he lost his legs he could no longer play sports. That was what he was told at any rate, but he would not give up. He found a sport, golf, that he could manage and he became a good golfer. His disability prevented him from taking part in what he had been good at before so he changed direction. He found a new sport that satisfied him and that he could manage. He did not give up. He gave up only what he could not do physically. He went in a different direction.

This is a very significant lesson for us all.

I am not saying it is easy because it is not. For most people, making changes in their life affects others beside themselves—family, friends and even work colleagues. You have to take them into consideration of course, but in the end the important thing is how well you can cope now that you have a hearing loss. It is not very helpful if you resist a change in your lifestyle, for example because it might affect your family, when you cannot cope yourself.

There are many things you will find more difficult than before, but there are also ways you can get round the difficulties or find new activities and ways of coping. For example, if you enjoyed music, you may not get the same enjoyment from it as you did in the past. However, if you listen to music with which you are familiar you can rely on your memory to fill in the bits that you do not get, although listening to new music can be very difficult. Another way you can get quite a lot of enjoyment from music is by watching ballet, which is motion put to music, and thus can be followed far more easily.

Going to the theatre

Although going to the theatre is not the same when you cannot hear properly, if you carefully plan your visit, there is still plenty there to enjoy. One of the problems is that with a hearing loss, it is difficult to pinpoint sound so that you do not know who is speaking. With a stage full of people, it is hard to pick out the person who is actually speaking. If you choose plays with only a few actors, it makes it far easier. For example, *Sleuth* has only two characters.

Another good idea is to read the play beforehand. This gives you a far better idea of what is going on when you get to the theatre. The Irish Hard of Hearing Association has play-reading nights for this purpose and then the group all go off to the theatre together and have a great time.

I know I watch other parts of the play

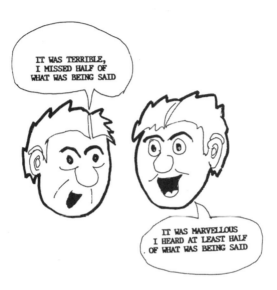

now. I particularly watch actors who are not speaking. This can be very interesting. The sets also can take on more interest and you can see how sets and props are used by the actors and are all part of the action as a whole.

Another thing to watch out for is mime—it can be wonderful and of course there are no words to worry about. Mime can be stimulating as well as funny and you will miss nothing.

The Abbey Theatre in Dublin occasionally puts on a special performances of a play with a caption board showing what the actors are saying. Watch out for these. The *Hearsay* magazine, the magazine of the Irish Hard of Hearing Association, sometimes has notification of these programmes.

Going out to dinner

Going out to dinner in a restaurant with a group can be most disturbing and difficult. It is essential that you do not just give up because if you do you will be denying yourself great pleasure. But do take a little care. Once again the trick is to watch where you are going. Some restaurants have tables very close together and noise from people talking and laughing can be magnified because they are so close. Watch out for carpets, curtains, glass and mirrors and even fountains. I had to change my table in a Chinese restaurant once because I was put right beside a small decorative fountain. The noise of the water falling drowned the speech. Nobody else was worried, but my hearing aid picked up the background noise of the water. Mirrors and windows can reflect back unwanted sound as well and it is better to avoid sitting in front of them if possible.

When you get to your chosen restaurant, watch where you sit. Look for overhead speakers because the piped music can get louder as time goes by. A table beside the

Getting on with life

Make up your mind to stop worrying about your hearing loss and to start thinking about everything else in your life. Hearing is only one of your senses. I do know how difficult and depressing a hearing loss can be. I have one myself. Our aim should be to get on with life and everything it throws at us.

I once went to the theatre with another hard of hearing person. When we came out at the end he said to me 'That was terrible. I missed half of what was going on.' I replied 'I thought it was great. I heard almost half of what was going on.' You see, it's the way you look at things that counts. Think about it.

door to the service area can be noisy and there can be a continual clatter of crockery and cutlery.

Be sure to tell others about your difficulty. If everyone else knows about your hearing loss, they can help. On one occasion, I went to a wedding reception and the hostess knew about my hearing difficulties and that I could hear better on the left-hand side. She especially seated me at the right-hand end of a table so that I could hear and also there was nobody on my right-hand side. She was able to do this because she knew about my hearing loss. Tell people and you will be surprised how thoughtful they can be.

Lip-reading

If you can, try to join up with a lip-reading class or group. Don't worry about not being able to hear because nobody else can either and you are all in the same boat. Not only will you learn things that are useful to you, you will also meet others who share your problems and difficulties. You will find out how other people cope and can tell others what you do as well.

You all learn from one another.

These classes are sometimes called 'aural rehabilitation'. I do not like the name myself as it always seems to need some explanation, whereas lip-reading seems self explanatory. Apparently, the idea is that more than lip-reading is involved, there are associated skills that will help those with a hearing loss. These include listening and communication skills and assertiveness.

Those who have to suffer our hearing loss along with us, our families for example, are also involved. Although we have the loss, our immediate families have to live with us; it is not easy for them either and it can be very frustrating for them. It is helpful if they are aware of what they can do to make communications generally easier. These can be quite simple things but they are not always understood or remembered (see pages 104–8).

However, don't think that you will go along for a few lessons and then be able to lip-read expertly because in all probability you will not. The main problem is that lip-reading is not an exact art. Lip shapes can sometimes be interpreted as saying different things. It is necessary to be fully aware of the context in which things are said in order to understand. But you will learn many things and it will certainly help you in your communications and confidence.

These groups are not all just hard work—in my experience there is usually quite a lot of fun as well. Some groups even stay together when the classes finish so that they can still meet and learn from one another. One group I know, which started from a lip-reading course, has been meeting now for over six years and is still going strong. One man in the group left and went to live in Wexford and the group still visits him in a body once or twice a year and makes an outing of it. Remember, it is far more difficult to cope with a hearing loss on your own, and certainly there is no need to.

Meetings/AGMs

All AGMs are rather similar; there is always the normal business to get through and the election of officers and then usually an open forum where anyone can bring up anything they like. At the Irish Hard of Hearing Association we always end up with a cup of tea or coffee and a biscuit, and we circulate and generally make people feel at home and listen to their problems. Many people come along, some old reliables, and some people who have never been before.

After this year's event, I got a letter from a man who had been to our AGM for the first time. He told me that he had been very apprehensive and expected everyone to be all doom and gloom, complaining of their hearing loss and being miserable generally. He was amazed at how well we all coped and, on the whole everyone was cheerful and enjoying themselves and circulating afterwards. It was an eye-opener for him because he had been trying to cope on his own up to that point. He could see just how much benefit there was from being able to talk about and share problems or even ambitions.

Many people avoid meetings like that and complain, without ever having been at any of them, that they would not be able to hear. In fact, at the IHHA AGM as well as the normal amplification system with microphones, there is a loop system (see page 128) and speed-text. This is a large screen where everything that is said comes up in writing so that everyone knows just what is going on. There is no excuse for not going because you think you will not know what is happening. You might even learn something about yourself. I am not suggesting that all meetings are like that because they are not but most hard of hearing meetings take into account that people find it difficult to hear.

Work and a hearing loss

For many of us our work is our lifeline. We do not want to jeopardise our jobs because of our hearing loss. I know so many hard of hearing people who are terrified that others will know that they have a hearing loss. They feel that if their boss finds out that they cannot hear properly, their job may well be on the line. This is very understandable, of course, and nobody wants to risk losing their bread and butter.

People in this kind of position are in a dilemma. Of course they must hold on to their jobs for as long as possible. They should certainly consider getting and wearing a hearing aid. Sometimes a hearing loss is more noticeabe than a hearing aid. That is well worth thinking about. Others do notice if you miss things. An aid may be so small that it is virtually invisible in the ear and hidden by the hair. One person I knew in business for nearly twenty years was quite shocked when I told him that I was wearing a hearing aid. He had never noticed at all over all those years.

A hearing aid may not always help enough for you to be able to carry on your job. It may be adequate for everyday normal life but not for work. For example, telephone operators or receptionists may find it extremely difficult to hear people's names and telephone numbers on the telephone. I know I find it very draining and even embarrassing at times. Sometimes, I can be talking to someone on the telephone for ten minutes before I gather just who it is, from something that they say. Teachers in a classroom may not be able to cope with the noise of pupils and what they say at the same time. Barristers may not hear the evidence or statements in court if their hearing is impaired.

There are some jobs, then, that need full hearing. There are others where it is not so important. Even still, many people will not disclose their hearing loss. One lady I knew did everything to cover up her hearing loss and eventually resigned before anyone found out. She then went on to do a degree course at university and ended up with a more suitable job. The new job was obtained when she had her loss and it was not necessary to try to hide it. She ended up with a much more rewarding job, having made a complete change of direction. It can be done. Another man, a barrister, gave up his job and became a solicitor instead, because of his hearing loss.

It is essential to think very carefully about the work you do and whether it is causing you distress or strain because of your hearing. Sometimes, by owning up to your loss it is possible to get a

change made in your work practice or
to get equipment that will help you to
cope. A telephonist may get an amplified
telephone, for example. One man I met
was in a semi-state organisation and
because of his hearing loss, retired early.
After joining the Irish Hard of Hearing
Association he learned about some of the
equipment that was available. He told me
that if he had known about these things
beforehand, he would not have retired at
all. Try to find out if there are things that
will help you before you make any drastic
changes. Maybe changes are not needed,
at the moment at any rate. A selection of
some of the aids available are detailed in
Chapter 7.

A change of direction or of your style
of work does not necessarily mean
downgrading. It can even mean going
into something more satisfying. It
could be a wonderful opportunity of
doing something different. It does not
necessarily mean the end, but can even
mean the beginning. Of course, it is not
given to everyone to be able to make big
changes in their lives. Going to university

is just not on for many people and even the Open University can be daunting, and expensive as well.

New interests can be opened up by going to evening classes. You may well be put off because you think you will not be able to hear. Do try anyway. Be sure to tell the instructor or lecturer that you have a hearing loss. They can be very helpful and even sometimes let you have notes of what they are saying if you ask nicely. Be sure to sit in the front row to get the best chance of hearing. Not all evening classes would be suitable but if you make careful enquiries, you may well find something that interests you.

Pitch and putt, golf

Changes do not have to be vast and even small alterations to the way you run your life can be helpful and remove anxiety. These do not have to be related to the work you do but to the life you lead. Some pastimes are ideal for the hard of hearing. Pitch and putt or golf can open up new vistas for you, if you are not already indoctrinated. Pitch and putt is inexpensive, good exercise and quiet. A good companion who understands is all you need. In fact you can even do it on your own, but some company helps to make the time so much more enjoyable.

If you want to go into golf more seriously you may well be put off by the expense of the whole thing. It is not the cost of the golf clubs that is the problem but the cost of joining a club, even if you can get in. However, there are many golfing societies that are not expensive and you will make many new friends when you join.

Flea powder

I popped my head around the corner of the door and said 'Did you see the back door keys ?'

My wife replied, 'No, I never noticed, but I'll get some powder for them when I'm out this afternoon.'

'What do you mean—get some powder for them?'

'Flea powder for the cat's fleas of course.'

7 Some useful equipment and ideas

Since I started to lose my hearing almost forty years ago, there have been many changes. Aids have got better and smaller, and equipment to help people to cope in a better way has been developed and improved enormously. No longer do I have to use an alarm clock in a biscuit tin to be able to get up on time in the morning. There are special clocks available now that do the job much better.

Texting on mobile phones

For the hard of hearing person, the mobile phone is one of the greatest inventions. We can communicate with others by text. Texting can be fast and good fun. You can keep in touch without the strain of having to listen. Your mobile can be used even if you are abroad and you can send back messages and receive bulletins from

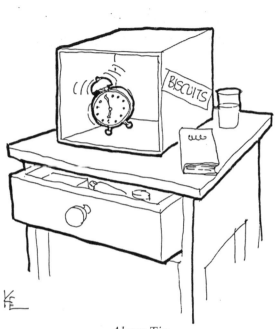

Alarm Tin

home while you are away. Many people are afraid of them and think they will not be able to use them properly. Don't be scared of them, they are really quite friendly. Get someone with a little patience to show you how to text messages and you will be in business very quickly. In fact you may wonder why you never got into texting before.

If you have the more expensive camera phones you can send photographs or pictures as well. Of course, it may well be that you can also hear on the mobile. I am not good at this, but in an emergency, I can just about hear on mine by holding it up to my aid, not my ear. I would not recommend it to anyone, but it is a possibility as the last resort. One of the great things about the mobile is that there is a range of prices to suit most pockets. Even for the senior citizen, you do not have to run up large bills but can top up your mobile whenever you like.

Telephones

I have said it before and I will say it many times again: 'I hate telephones.' I hear the telephone bell going and I shudder. Many people speak badly or quickly on the telephone and I just cannot make them out. When it comes to addresses or numbers, I am completely lost. I use a special hands-free telephone which speaks out into the room and I should be able to hear all right, but for some reason, I just cannot. Nevertheless, there are many different telephones out and one of them may help you.

Most telephones have a built-in inductive coupler fitted into the earpiece. This means that if you use the T switch on your hearing aid, you should be able to hear the incoming speech perfectly. Of course, you will not be able to hear what you are saying yourself. That can be a bit of a snag for some people. There are also amplified telephones which make it possible for you to increase or decrease the volume to what you need. In this way, incoming speech can be heard more clearly. The dB30 phone is excellent; it has an extra-loud ringing sound, has large buttons, is hearing aid compatible, and an illuminated call indicator which lights up when the phone rings.

All these telephones are available from Eircom.

Telephone/fax machines

One piece of equipment that I find excellent is the combined telephone and fax. It is a little larger than an ordinary telephone and there are several makes. Some take A4 paper to print out messages and others take paper rolls. The great thing about these is that you need no typing skills to use them. If you want to you can just write out a message by hand and send it off or even send a newspaper clipping or a photograph. One drawback is that the quality of illustrations is poor, not like email and will only come out in black and white. And of course you can only send faxes to someone who also has a fax machine.

All you have to do is to buy the machine and plug it into an electric socket and also into a telephone point and it is as simple as that. You do not have to switch it on and it works away even if you are not there and takes your messages. It is a great way of keeping in touch.

Email and the Internet

Although texting is excellent for the hard of hearing, computers can offer even more help to those with a hearing loss. There is a very definite limit to what it is possible to do with texting, but with the Internet it is easy to get all sorts of information without having to strain to hear.

Getting dates, prices or times of events, for example, cannot be achieved with texting but most events now supply website addresses and you can get all the information from them. There are websites for almost everything—for items for sale, general information, train timetables, entertainment—the list is endless.

If you have an email address you can communicate with so many of your friends and even send them photographs or recipes. They can send you messages, and there is no problem with trying to hear as would be the case on the telephone. You do not even have to answer the email immediately but can reply in your own good time, just as you would by ordinary post.

It is well worth the effort to learn to use computers, to be connected to the Internet and use email. Many people are afraid of computers but with just a little effort , it is surprising just how easy it is to learn enough to make life so much easier for yourself. We all complain that having a hearing loss limits our communication skills, but using a computer opens up almost limitless possibilities and all without the hassle, effort and strain of trying to hear.

Television and radio

For many people who are hard of hearing, the television is great but even the old radio can be enjoyed. If you are buying either, do be sure that you get a remote control. This is simply magic—you can turn the volume up if people are whispering or the music has become very low and just as quickly turn it back down when the sound is restored to its normal level. This can all be done from your chair without fuss and if someone says something to you, you can turn down the volume and you are not completely cut off from others. If you are playing a CD or a DVD, you can even use the pause button so that you do not lose out on anything.

Television texting

It can be helpful to get a television that shows texting. I find it is essential. By pressing the text button on the remote control and keying in 888, texting comes up at the bottom of the screen and tells you what people are actually saying. It is not perfect by any means—sometimes there is a time lag when people say something and the text follows a little later. In some programmes, those that have been pre-recorded, you may well find that the texting comes up before the person actually speaks.

Not all programmes have texting but thanks to a lot of hard work by a few dedicated people, there is about 80 per cent texting of programmes on the major channels. Some of the channels do no texting at all. On the whole, texting is very good and allows us to enjoy films, news and even sport, and know what is going on. The texting may not always be as good as it should be and sometimes there are dreadful mistakes, but on the whole it is good and certainly I personally could not enjoy television without it.

The Irish Hard of Hearing Association has its own page on RTE Aertel. By pressing the text button and putting in 494 the page comes up on the screen with up-to-date information and news of forthcoming social events. This initiative is only in its infancy and it is hoped to develop it to give more information as time goes by.

Infra red listening devices

There are now several TV and radio listening devices available. These are based on an infra-red system. The sound from your TV or radio is channelled through a transmitter by an infra-red signal which is picked up by a small receiver which is part of a headset or neck loop. The Infraport 810 is supplied with a headset which is comfortable to wear . The user can move about for up to 12 metres and adjust the incoming volume without disturbing anyone else in the room at the time. The battery is recharged simply by replacing the headset on its transmitter.

The Infraport 810s has a neck loop and is used with the T switch on your hearing aid. Sound is directed straight into your hearing aid and once again it is possible to adjust the volume. There are other forms of systems available—you can see some of them at DeafTech in South Frederick Street, Dublin (see Chapter 10).

Loop systems

Many people are a little baffled by loop systems. They just do not know what they are and what they do. Very simply, a loop of wire is taken around a certain area and coupled up to a booster and a microphone. Voices and sounds are converted into electrical pulses and sent around the wire loop. If you are inside the loop and have a T switch on your hearing aid, you should be able to hear what is being said, or what sounds are being produced, without any background noise. Very roughly, that is a non-technical description of what happens.

However, things are not quite as simple as that in practice. If the system is working properly, you will hear all right but you will not hear anything else. For example, in a theatre, you might be able to hear what is being said on stage, but you will not hear any comments from your friend in the seat beside you. You will be cut off completely from everything but what is on the loop. Many people, myself included, do not like this very much. Another problem is that you must keep fairly still. If you move your head, even up and down a little, the volume of the sound you hear can vary.

The worst problem is that the majority of those installing loop systems seem to have perfect hearing. They can only test the system by using a hearing aid in the hand. If it squeaks, they think, the system must work. This is not the case at all. Many of the systems installed just do not work. Only those with a hearing loss and wearing an aid with a T switch can properly test them.

In addition, loops are not always installed in the right positions and in some cases are fitted in the most convenient places rather than the best places. For example, in one theatre, the loop was fitted at a very high ceiling level around the theatre. It was too far away from the seating and it was impossible to hear anything from any position in the auditorium. The installer thought it was perfect and so did the management, but it was useless for those with a hearing loss.

Some loop systems work very well indeed and there are many churches, for example, where the system works perfectly. One difficulty is that even if the system works well, those in charge of using it may not be familiar enough with it. Sometimes it is not switched on at all. One priest does not use the loop installed in his church because he believes his voice is very strong and can be heard perfectly in all parts of the church. That kind of thing is very sad and it is obvious that the hard of hearing are not getting their message across very well.

There are also small loop systems installed for very local conditions, for example in post offices. You will recognise these by the ear symbol with the diagonal bar through it. If you want to use one of these, you may well have to ask for it to be switched on. The counter staff are not always conversant with the system.

You will also see signs for loop systems in the various airports. If you stand under one of these signs and turn on your T switch, you should be able to hear announcements. Once again, you will not hear anything or anyone else.

Flashing signals

It is all very well having telephones and door bells in your home but can you hear if they are ringing? It is great being able to hear on the telephone, but do you know if it is ringing? Are your friends standing in the street ringing the front door bell and you do not hear them? Of course, it happens all the time. Once again modern technology has come up with the answer.

In my own home, I have a system called the Universal Visual Warning. There are four orange lights which can be fitted anywhere in the house so that wherever you are, you can see one of them. They are connected to a distribution box and to the telephone and the front door bell. When the telephone rings, the orange lights pulsate and when the door bell goes, the light comes on for about a minute and then goes off again. It is magic. The only problem is that the entire thing has to be wired up and it is quite complicated. But once installed, it is fantastic. Mine has been going strong for about fifteen years now without any problems.

There are now more modern systems that do not need the same amount of installation. Once again DeafTech has these on display. If you live in the country, try to make a visit to Dublin to see them. Your journey could be well worth while, and you may keep your friends from standing out in the cold for hours on end.

Hearing dogs

For some people, a hearing dog can be of great help. These dogs are trained to tell you when a telephone is ringing or if the front door bell is going. Hearing dogs are not for everyone—both dog and user have to be trained and it takes time and effort. You cannot just go out and buy a hearing dog.

Alarm clocks

Of course you take your aids out when you go to bed but without them you will not be able to hear the average alarm clock. Vibrating pads are great. They go under the pillow and are attached by a wire to a special alarm clock. At the appropriate time, the clock sets the pad vibrating under your pillow and wakes you up. I have one of these, but once, unknown to me, the pad slipped down behind the bed and in the morning I woke up to hear a banging on the front door. The neighbours thought our boiler was about to burst with the dreadful rattling noise. What had happened was that the vibrator rattled between the party wall and the bed-head. It did not disturb me, or anyone else in the house, but it terrified the neighbours. I have now safety-pinned the wire holding the vibrator to the sheets to stop it travelling. I have also upgraded the system so that now a light comes on at the same time as the pad vibrates so that one or the other wakes me up. There are several types of this alarm clock available. DeafTech have some on view.

There is also a kind of travel alarm clock which you set and put under the pillow. The whole clock vibrates at the set time. However, if your hearing is very bad like mine, it may not be strong enough to wake you.

Smoke alarms

These are so important but the normal ones only make a sound so at night they are useless for the hard of hearing, with hearing aids taken out. There are special smoke alarms made for the hard of hearing which light up when activated. Once again, DeafTech has them on display.These are just a few of the many items now available on the market. Ask around about other items and do ask your hearing aid supplier who will probably be more conversant with what is available. Things are changing all the time and new products are being invented and introduced.

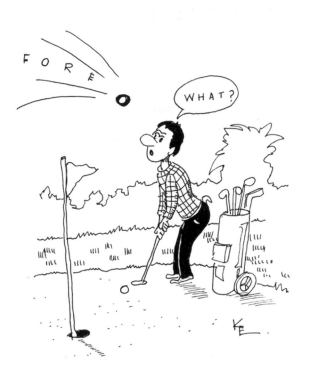

8 Helpful tips

One of the major difficulties with having a hearing loss is that you try to hear everything. If you are out in a group, don't be afraid to sit back and let some things go. Much of what people say is rubbish anyway. Nearly fifty per cent will be repetition or embellishment. That means you only have to catch fifty per cent and you will know what is going on.

Straining to hear all the time is exhausting and after an hour or two you will be worn out. Ordinary hearing people are not under the same strain. They can talk for hours, very often with meaningless conversation, and it has no effect on them at all. It is not the same for us. This is particularly so if there is loud background noise. We have to strain extra hard to catch words over the loud background sounds. The more you turn up your hearing aid, the worse the background noise becomes.

I have found that in situations like this, I turn my hearing aid volume down a little. This reduces everything but it does make speech a little clearer.

On one occasion, a group of us went out to a pub. We were all hard of hearing and the noise was tremendous. We all turned off our aids and attempted to converse. It was hilarious. We have all tried to learn lip reading and we are all very bad at it and you can imagine how much we got wrong. The main thing was that we were all in the same boat. We all had the same disability. Nobody looked a fool because we were all the same. The tears came to our eyes because we were laughing so much. We ended up having a wonderful time. Who said you can't go out and enjoy yourself because you have a hearing loss?

Having said this, be a little cautious. It is a bad idea to be with hard of hearing people all the time. After all, we belong to the hearing world and we have to cope in that situation. In the Irish Hard of Hearing Association, we hold many social meetings such as hill walking, music nights, play reading, seminars and so on.

We always have hearing people there as well. This gives a better balance and it also helps the normal hearing people to understand our needs a little better. It is important not to hide away in a little world of your own even if it is comfortable and less demanding.

When you are tired, your hearing may get worse. That is why it is essential not to strain all the time to hear everything. I just switch off at the most unlikely times. Walking down the street I don't need to hear anyone so I switch off and all the traffic noises just evaporate. It's magic, really. When I meet a certain friend of mine in the street, I know she has switched off as well because the first thing she does is to put her finger to her ear to switch on again and, of course, I do the same.

Stress and fatigue can affect your hearing. This does not mean that if you eliminate stress and get plenty of sleep your hearing will get better. It just does not work that way. It does mean that what little hearing you have can be badly affected if you are tired and strained, and you should do anything you can to reduce stress.

[97]

Relaxation can help your hearing. But don't get me wrong. It doesn't make your hearing any better, but it can give you the best chance of hearing. Things like Yoga and Tsai Chi are excellent and can be readily enjoyed by those who suffer from a hearing loss. Do try to find something that suits you and can help you to relax. But if you attend classes you need to choose carefully—it will not help you very much if you have to strain all the time to hear what is going on.

It may sound weird but there's actual hard evidence that exercise can improve your hearing. Scientists say that it happens because regular exercise increases the blood circulation to the inner ear which, in turn, enhances your powers of hearing. This does not mean that you have to go down to the gym and do push-ups or run for miles on a moving platform. There is nothing better than just walking, although I don't mean just one turn around the block. A decent walk of several miles in the fresh air is excellent, particularly if it is regular and not just a one off.

There are a number of specific things

people with a hearing loss can do to help themselves in social situations. With just a little bit of thought, it is possible to improve things for ourselves and make it easier for others to help us as well. Before, we used to be able to go anywhere and do anything without giving it a thought. Now, it is essential to think about these things beforehand so that it eases things for us.

How to help yourself

Give yourself the best possible chance to hear what the other person is saying.

Make sure you are squarely facing the person and are no more than three to four feet away and of course, on the same level. If the person speaking to you is sitting down, you should be sitting down as well.

Try to avoid group activities. It is difficult to know what one person is saying but when it comes to a group, it is nearly impossible. It is difficult even to know who is speaking.

Some time ago, I had to visit a factory and was brought into a very noisy area where the manager started to tell me about the work going on. After a while, I noticed that we were tending to go around in circles and I asked him if he had a hearing loss. He told me he had. We had each been spending the last ten minutes trying to get the other person on our good side. Once we knew we were both hard of hearing, we left the noisy area and were able to do business over a cup of coffee in a quiet canteen. If you tell other people about your hearing loss, they can often help you.

If you are invited to a party, do not just turn down the invitation because you think you will not be able to cope. Go, but take a little care. Try not to sit down and become a permanent fixture. If you are standing, you can easily move on if you cannot hear the person beside you if they speak badly or mumble. Avoid men with moustaches or beards because their mouths are too well insulated for you to see what they are saying. Keep away from high reflecting surfaces like mirrors or windows and take up your position in a corner. Look out for surfaces that will absorb sound, like heavy curtains or carpets or upholstery. A corner can be a good place to stand because any sound reflection bounces off at an angle and not directly at you. Avoid the centre of the room because people will be talking all around you and you will hear nothing but background noise.

Watch out for lighting, both natural and artificial. Be sure that you have your back to the light source so that the face of the person speaking is well illuminated. Do be careful not to stand in front of the window because although it gives good light on the speaker's face there is excessive sound reflection.

It is so important to be able to see who is talking. Even if you do not lip read, a person's lips and expressions can tell you quite a lot.

Many places these days have background sound, live music for example. Watch out for speakers so that you can keep away from them. Most background music is far too loud, even for normal hearing people. Natural features, like small fountains, also can obliterate sound. I have had to move my seat in a restaurant because of a near-by fountain. When I moved, I could hear much better. Remember, even a simple thing like a piano, which may be perfectly all right when nobody is sitting at it, can be dreadful when someone comes along and starts to play. Once again, in a restaurant, I had to change my seat. When I went in, there was no one at the piano, but half way through the meal someone came along and started to play. It was a disaster and I could not hear a thing. The pianist was very upset.

Background noise is deadly if you are wearing a hearing aid. If you visit a friend at their home, be sure to ask them to turn the TV off or the radio down. They will be used to this continual noise and can ignore it, but you are not able to do that. Another friend of mine always has his car radio on and when I am sitting beside him and he is driving, he is on my wrong side to start with and the radio blots out what he is saying. I always have to remind him to turn off the radio and every time he completely forgets. I did ask him to turn the radio off once only to discover that he was actually talking on the telephone and I did not realise it. He thought it was very funny.

If you go to the theatre, choose your play carefully. Try to go to plays that have few actors in it. Experiment with things that have no speaking, mime and dance, for example. Perhaps you never went to anything like this before, but it may well open up new doors for you and you may enjoy them enormously. You certainly will not have any difficulty in hearing, because nothing is said anyway. If you go to a concert, try to sit on the side of the theatre that the violins are on, that is, on the left hand side. The heavier instruments will be on the right. It all helps, especially if you are in the front row. In the National Concert Hall in Dublin, there is a balcony around the back of the stage. If you sit there, you will be immediately over the timpani and it can be difficult to hear the rest of the orchestra. Incidentally, the National Concert Hall has an excellent loop system.

How others can help

Now let us look at how others can help us. The first thing, of course, is that other people must know that you have a hearing problem so do tell them if you want them to accommodate you. Once they know, there are many things that are helpful and will make things easier for you.

Some of those are things we have covered already. People must face you and have the light on their faces so that you can see them properly. If they know which is your best side, they can be sure to stand on that side if they want to communicate with you. This sounds obvious, but it is amazing how many people just do not realise how helpful it can be. These small things make all the difference in the world.

Do not forget that you have a hidden disability. To look at you others would not know about your hearing loss. It is not like other disabilities, most of which are visually apparent. With a hearing loss, you look the same as normal hearing people and others either do not know or even forget very quickly. I have a friend who always remembers about my hearing loss. She makes sure that she is on my better side and if we are out with a group of people for a meal, makes sure that I have a seat at the end of the table so that I only have people talking on my good side. It is helpful and considerate.

When people know about your loss, they tend to shout at you so that you will be able to hear. This does not help at all so be sure to tell them to speak normally but clearly. Most people have no idea what it is like to have a hearing loss and they never will unless you tell them. It is not necessary to keep on at them because you will just bore them to tears. A casual reminder every now and then does wonders, though.

When people are speaking to you, it is far easier to hear sentences rather than just single words. Encourage them in this and if you do not hear them, get them to say it another way, this can often help. There can be a little time lag sometimes before you work out just what someone has said. This is quite normal.

Someone speaking to you should not

bob their head around or turn it frequently. Constant movement of the head can make it very difficult for someone with a hearing loss to hear the speaker. The speaker's mouth should be seen at all times. How many times have you had friends speaking with their hands in front of their mouths, or smoking or even eating? It is difficult enough to hear without this added encumbrance as well. The last straw is chewing gum. You will not know if the person is speaking or chewing.

It is always a good idea to make others aware of your hearing difficulties. Mind you it can sometimes have comical results. I was making a visit to the local hospital and had to wait for ages. The room was full of patients and I had to sit at the back. When the nurse came around and collected our pink cards I told her I had a problem and asked her to be sure to make sure I heard her when she called me. After half an hour the front seats emptied so I moved up so that I could hear better. Shortly afterwards the nurse came back and shouted at the top of her voice 'KENNETH EDWARDS'. It startled everyone. Books and magazines tumbled to the floor and people shifted in their seats and woke up. Suddenly the place seemed alive with activity. I stood up and tapped the nurse on the shoulder and said 'Here I am'. She had thought I was still at the back of the room.

All this is important, but of course, if the hard of hearing person is not aware someone is trying to communicate with them, it is all a waste of time. Attract the person's attention before trying to say anything. This is a very important point. I have fallen into this trap myself very often simply because I do not think. Sometimes when my wife, who has a hearing loss as well, is working at the sink or somewhere else with her back to me, I say something to her and she has no idea I am even speaking. When I get no answer from her, I remember and have to tap her on the shoulder and start again. It is so easy to forget.

Sometimes gestures are excellent in making a sentence easier to interpret. There are so many things that are almost self explanatory. A wink or a smile or a nod and hand movements and gestures all help to reinforce the sentence. Fingers can be used to interpret numbers, and of course these are so difficult to hear and easy to get wrong. One hard of hearing person I know is trying to learn sign language. I queried her about this because few other people who are not deaf learn it and she would not be able to use it very much. Then she told me that two of her family were also going to classes with her. She thinks it will make things at home much easier. That's quite a thought.

It is always so helpful if a hard of hearing person knows what you are talking about. In normal conversation, the subject matter can change quickly and even several times and it leaves the listener floundering, unless someone lets them know that the subject has moved on.

All of these tips are important and are especially good with people you know well and spend a lot of of time with, like family or workmates. Over a period of time they can learn what is helpful for you. However, we do not always know the people we are talking to and they may well be complete strangers. It is more difficult to tell people you do not know what you need, people in shops or in the street or in the hairdressers for example. When I go to get my hair cut, I always go to the same place and the same person. I always explain exactly what I want before I take my aids out because when they are out I just can't hear a thing. Over the years the barber has learnt what I want and he is very understanding but sometimes he forgets as well and says something.

Travelling

Travelling can be difficult, especially by air. It is important to be on the watch all the time. You can see from the announcement board what gate your departure is from, but you might well miss an announcement if there is a change. This has happened to me on more than one occasion. It is only by watching the other travellers that you can find out if something unusual is happening. If they start running away from your gate, you can be sure they have heard something you missed. Just follow them and hope for the best, don't hang around.

Helpful tips

I was told by a friend of mine that when she checked in at the airport, she showed them a little badge she had which said 'Hard of Hearing—Please Speak Clearly'. When it came to the boarding time, she was taken on board before anyone else. I suppose they wanted to know where she was sitting in case there was an emergency.

When you finally get to your holiday hotel, tell the staff that you have a hearing loss. This is important. If there is a fire, you might be left behind. It is just conceivable that you will not hear a fire alarm call. I know one hard of hearing person who was in a hotel in England and was awakened when a large burly fireman burst the door down. She had not heard the alarm going off. Luckily the staff knew she was hard of hearing. We are very vulnerable when we have taken our hearing aids out.

One nice thing about holidays abroad is that you have become more equal with most other tourists. When a foreign language is spoken, most visitors do not know what is being said so that your hearing is not so important anyway.

[110]

If you are on holidays and you go down to the beach, what do you do with your hearing aids when you want to swim? If you take them out and just leave them under something, they are prone to get sand into them, or you might even walk on them. One answer is to get one of those waterproof containers that hang around your neck, usually to keep money in. However, this can easily be stolen. I have bought myself a large brimmed hat with tiny useless pockets in the crown. It is excellent to keep me out of the sun and when I go in for a swim I put my aids in the little pockets. There they are perfectly safe and dry.

Everywhere you go, be sure you have a packet of spare batteries. You never know just when you are going to go off the air. When I go on holidays, I also always take a spare old aid and an ear mould. If anything goes wrong, I have some kind of spare even if it is not as good as my current aid, it is far better than nothing.

When you have a hearing problem you find that you have certain options that normal people do not have. For example, when you are in a very noisy place, maybe children are yelling all around you, just switch off. You will find the peace delicious. I switch off quite frequently and find it very calming and relaxing. Anywhere I can, in noisy places or busy streets, I turn off. It is so easy and if you meet someone you know, it is so simple to just switch on again.

At the lip-reading class
The lip-reading class was discussing relaxation. Someone happened to mention 'smelling salts'. One man innocently asked what smelly socks had got to do with relaxation? There was silence for a moment, and then the penny dropped and everyone burst out laughing.

9 Living with some-one with a hearing loss

Half the time we seem to think that we have the option on misery. We are the ones who have to suffer our hearing loss. We are the ones who cannot hear. Make no mistake about it, others have to suffer our loss as well, particularly those who live with us or work with us. We all know how bad our communications with others have become, but those close to us also have these difficulties.

Making a quick comment as in the past now becomes a much more laboured exercise. The sort of thing I mean is when your spouse turns to you and remarks, for example, 'This is a terrible programme'.

Of course, the remark is so sudden that you don't catch it and you reply 'What ?' Your spouse repeats the remark and you say 'I didn't think it was incredible.'

'No, I said it was terrible, not incredible.'

'What was that again?'

'Oh never mind, it doesn't matter.'

You see what I mean; perfectly normal little remarks become big deals. Without a doubt, it is extremely frustrating and difficult for people with normal hearing to fully realise what you are going through, but it is also very difficult for you to fully realise just how difficult it is for others. Once, someone I was speaking to got very cross and started to shout at me. They just could not understand that I could not hear what they were saying.

This is why it is so important to tell people you have difficulty hearing. If you do not, they might well think you are just stupid and treat you as such. Your own family already know about your hearing problem but that does not make it any easier for them.

This chapter is meant for those who live with a person who has a hearing loss and much of what I am saying I have already mentioned. I make no apologies for this because it is very important for normal hearing people to know how to help us.

Of course, there are things that can be helpful to both parties. As I mentioned in the last chapter, it is essential to make sure that the person you are talking to knows you are about to say something. A quick nudge can alert the hard of hearing person that something is coming. This is most helpful.

If there are a good few people in the house, say around the dining-room table during a meal, it is very difficult for the person who is hard of hearing to know who is speaking. With a hearing loss, the ability to pinpoint the direction the sound is coming from is limited or even non-existent. If there are several people present, especially where quick short sentences or a word are concerned, the sound is gone before it is possible to catch who said it and it is too late to see whose lips were moving. It does take a little understanding and patience on both sides.

Another pitfall with families and at home is when something is said, but a noise is being produced at the same time.

A typical example of this is when the husband or wife is at the kitchen sink with the tap running and says something. The noise of the running water into the sink drowns out the words. Just turning off the tap for a moment works wonders. I am not being clever here and I must admit that my wife and I fall into little traps like this all the time even though we are aware of them.

At the same time, we do get it right half of the time. There are so many noisy machines around the house, such as the vacuum cleaner, the electric kettle, the dishwasher and the washing machine, to name just a few. All these create sounds that blot out the possibility of hearing speech, so do be careful. Incidentally, it is possible to get an electric kettle that makes very little noise when it starts to boil. And do not forget electric drills, electric screwdrivers, hedge clippers and so on. Remembering these things can make life a little easier for the hard of hearing person but at the same time it can save you so much frustration yourself.

One very big difficulty, especially for

husbands and wives, is entertainment. If one person likes the cinema or the pub or some similar kind of entertainment, this can be very hard for the partner with the hearing loss. This in itself can put a great strain on any marriage because it seems impossible to find pleasant things to do together.

It calls for a little give and take and it is useful to get together and talk it out—in a nice quiet atmosphere, of course. There may well be things that you can both enjoy without putting too much pressure on either person. You can both still enjoy a nice meal out, for example, if you choose your restaurant carefully. A noisy background can be disturbing. I know, I have been out at restaurants and the background music is terribly loud. I now ask if it is possible to turn it down a bit and sometimes they actually do so.

I did mention that someone shouted at me and believed that I would be able to hear what they were saying much better. Of course this is nonsense and actually makes it far more difficult. If you are speaking to someone with a hearing loss, it is far better to speak clearly in a normal voice and perhaps a little slower. Do avoid single words and if the person to whom you are speaking does not get what you are saying, try to say it another way. This can be very helpful. Very long sentences can also be difficult to understand, so do keep to short sentences if possible.

Whatever you do or say, try not to bob your head around but keep it relatively still and do not keep turning it backwards and forwards. If someone is trying to lip-read you they just cannot cope with this kind of thing. Remember to keep your hands away from your face and never speak with a cigarette in your mouth and avoid chewing gum like the plague. These tips sound pretty obvious but it is amazing how many people just do not think of them.

Another fallacy is that people need to exaggerate facial movements. This tends to distort lip movement and once again is not helpful particularly if someone is trying to lip-read you. Just speak normally, perhaps a little louder but not shouting.

One of my own disappointments is

with children, particularly with my grandchildren. They have lovely but indistinct voices. I could never hear what they were saying to me and I feel I have missed so much. Many children either mumble quietly or shout at you. I found that it was difficult to converse with them and I missed out on their childhood. I just could not be with them on my own. Now that they have grown up, I am able to converse with them quite normally. Teenagers, of course, have their own problems and they seem to have been weaned on loud noise. If they are in the house, there is music roaring away, filling the whole place. I do not know why, but music these days has to be at some extraordinary high level to be enjoyed.

Many people seem to think that because we cannot hear, we are also daft or stupid as well. Maybe they do not know how to speak to us or perhaps are afraid to in case we do not understand or make a fool of them. When a hard of hearing person is out with a normal hearing person it is very noticeable. For example in a shop, the attendant will speak to the normal hearing person almost as if the hard of hearing person were not there at all. The shop assistant, for instance, may say 'What size shoes does he take?' I must admit, if I hear this kind of thing I always reply directly back to the assistant 'I take size nine thank you.' Sometimes they seem quite surprised that I am able to speak at all. Maybe I'm exaggerating all this and am just a little sensitive. It is essential, however, not to ignore the hard of hearing person. It does little to help their self esteem, which can be rather low in the first place.

A really great help for me is when I am aware of the subject matter. I have mentioned this before and make no apologies for saying it again. I have a friend who always gives me the tip-off about what is being discussed. It is done in a simple and quiet way but it does mean that I have a much better chance of being able to follow the general conversation.

A final tip is always to carry a small notebook and pencil with you. If you need to give someone with a hearing loss an address or the name of a meeting place or time or telephone number, or something important, write it down for them, then there is some chance they will have it right. Do remember that for a person with a hearing loss, numbers are easy to get wrong.

Do's and don'ts when with a person with a hearing loss
• do speak clearly
• do tell the person the subject of the conversation
• do carry a notebook and pencil so you can write down details
• do speak clearly in a normal voice and perhaps a little more slowly
• do avoid single words and very long sentences
• do vary the way you say things if the person to whom you are speaking does not get what you are saying
• do make sure that there is light on your face
• don't exaggerate facial movements
• don't move your head or bob about
• don't cover your mouth
• don't shout
• don't smoke or chew gum

10 Further information

When you want help or advice, it is not always easy to find out where to go to get it. The following addresses may be helpful to get you started in the right direction.

Deafhear
Gives advice and help to both deaf and hard of hearing people throughout Ireland; runs local hearing help groups and support groups for lip-reading skills; publishes a magazine, *LINK*.

Deafhear resource centres:
Dublin city centre
35 North Frederick Street, Dublin 1
tel 01 817 5700 fax 01 878 3629
e-mail info@deafhear.ie ruth.mccullagh@deafhear.ie
Dublin south (Tallaght)
Unit G/H Exchange Hall. Belgard Square North, Tallaght, Dublin 24

tel 01 462 0377 fax 01 462 0378
text 086 171 6284
e-mail dublinsouth@deafhear.ie
Dundalk
Regional Sensory Resource Centre, 14 Jocelyn
St, Dundalk, Co.Louth
tel 042 933 2010 fax 042 938 9186
text 042 938 9186
e-mail dundalk@deafhear.ie
Galway
9a St Francis Street, Galway
tel 091 564 871 fax 091 564 873
text 086 864 8659
e-mail galway@deafhear.ie
Kilkenny
44 Friary Street, Kilkenny
tel 056 776 3508 fax 056 776 3782
e-mail kilkenny@deafhear.ie
Killarney
10 Flemings Lane, High Street, Killarney, Co.
Kerry
tel 064 6620052 fax 064 6620053 ie
text 086 805 6202
e-mail killarney@deafhear.
Letterkenny
Sensory Resource Centre, Justice Walshe
Road, Letterkenny, Co. Donegal
tel 074 918 8252 fax 074 918 8240
text 074 918 8240/086 885 8194
e-mail letterkenny@deafhear.ie

Further information

Limerick

1st floor, 4 Henry Street, Limerick
tel 061 467 494/5 fax 061 467 497
text 086 222 9638
e-mail limerick@deafhear.ie

Tullamore

Church Street. Tullamore. Co.Offaly
tel 057 935 1606 fax 057 932 6425
text 057 932 6421
e-mail tullamore@deafhear.ie

Waterford

Cheshire Home, John's Hill, Waterford
tel 051 855 777 fax 051 852 132
e-mail maureen.whittle@deafhear.ie

Wexford

Lochrann House, Cinema Lane, Wexford
tel 053 915 2645 fax 053 915 2646
text 053 915 2647
e-mail annie.murphy@deafhear.ie

Deafhear services can also be accessed
through extensive outreach programmes.
Contact your nearest Deafhear resource centre
for venues and times in your area.

DeafTech

35 North Frederick Street, Dublin 1
tel 01 872 3800 fax 01-878 3629
e-mail deafhear@iol.ie
Stocks and sells equipment and useful

gadgets suitable and helpful for the hard of hearing. Provides technical and non-technical information on deafness and hearing loss.

Disability Federation of Ireland
Fumbally Court, Fumbally Lane, Dublin 8
tel 01 454 7978

Friends of the Elderly
25 Bolton Street, Dublin 1
tel 01 873 1855 fax 01 873 1617
Volunteers visit lonely older people in their homes. Organises social activities in or from Bolton Street

Irish Association of Older People
4 Sussex Street, Dún Laoghaire, Co. Dublin
tel. 01 214 0737

Irish Hard of Hearing Association
35 North Frederick Street, Dublin 1
tel 01 872 3816 fax 01 872 3816 e-mail ihha@ deafhear.ie website www.ihha.ie
Gives advice and help with problems of dealing with a hearing loss and runs social events in the Dublin area.
Publishes a magazine *Hearsay.*

Irish Senior Citizens Parliament
90 Fairview Strand, Dublin 3

tel 01 856 1243
Represents 300 organisations of older and
retired people and represents their needs and
issues to the Government.

Irish Society of Hearing Aid Audiologists
(ISHAA)
website www.ishaa.ie

Irish Tinnitus Association
35 North Frederick Street, Dublin 1
tel 01 8723800 fax 01 8723816 text messages 01
878 3629 e-mail ita@deafhear.ie

RTE Aertel page 499
Special pages of information on television
accessed by the text button on the TV. Type in
888 to get sub-titles on programmes.

Glossary

Terms and expressions used in the hard of hearing world.

Audiogram Graph showing decibel readings for each ear recorded by the audiologist

Audiologist Professional trained to evaluate hearing loss and related disorders

Background noise Noise in the background that blots out immediate sound preventing it from being heard

Behind-the-ear aid Hearing aid that goes behind the ear, joined to the ear mould by tubing

Body aid Hearing aid worn on the body

Bone conduction Sound stimulating the inner ear directly, bypassing the outer and middle ear

Conductive hearing loss Hearing loss in the outer or middle ear

Decibels Measure of the amount of sound heard

Ear mould Plastic mould shaped to match the interior of the ear

Glossary

Ear wax Wax that builds up in the ear and can affect the hearing

ENT consultant Medical specialist dealing with problems of the ear, nose and throat

Feedback Whistling sound produced when air gets past the ear mould or there is a poor joint between tube and mould or aid

Glue ear Fluid behind the ear which prevents a child from hearing

Hard ear mould Ear mould made from hard plastic

In-the-canal aid Aid that fits into the canal of the ear

In-the-ear aid Aid that fits into the ear itself; larger than in-the-canal aid

Lip-reading Reading the pattern of lip movements during ordinary speech

Lip-speaking Speaking without sound by means of clear lip movement

Loop system Insulated wire connected to an amplifier and a microphone. A person within the looped area can hear by means of the T switch on their hearing aid.

Meniere's disease Disease of the inner ear that can result in vertigo, tinnitus and hearing loss

Residual hearing Hearing that a deaf child has

Sensorineural hearing loss Hearing loss in the inner ear

Soft ear mould Ear mould made from soft plastic

Glossary

Speed text Computer-aided note-taking recording what is said at meetings and projected on a screen so that people can read it

Texts Refers to texting on mobiles phones.

Tinnitus Noises heard in the head which do not come from outside the ear

T-switch Switch on hearing aid to enable sound to be heard by means of a loop system

Tube Plastic tube that connects the hearing aid to the ear mould.

Catholic churches with audio induction loop systems

Loop systems are installed in many churches and public buildings. They do not always work and sometimes they are not switched on. The following list of churches with loop systems was compiled by the Irish Hard of Hearing Association and comprises only those which responded to a general circular. There may be many more not listed or installed since this list was compiled.

If there is no loop system in your church, why not ask for one to be installed? It is only by asking that we achieve results.

Diocese of Armagh
Aughnacloy,Tyrone: St Mary's
Beragh, Tyrone: Immaculate Conception
Blackrock,Dundalk: St Oliver Plunkett
Bridge St, Dundalk: St Nicholas'
Cathedral Rd, Armagh: St Patrick's Cathedral
Coalisland,Tyrone: SS Mary & Joseph

Cullyhanna, Armagh: St Patrick's
Darvey, Louth: St Michael's
Dromiskin, Louth: St Peter's
Drumalane, Newry: St Mary of the
   Assumption
Dungannon, Tyrone: St Patrick's
Dunleer, Louth: St Brigid's
Dunmoyle, Ballgawley: St Mary's
Haggardstown, Dundalk: St Fursey's
Keedy, Armagh: St Patrick's
Kilkerley: Immaculate Conception
Killeenan, Kildress: St Joseph's
Lissan, Tyrone: St Michael's
Moneymore, Derry: SS John & Trea
Moorstown, Ardboe: Immaculate Conception
Moy, Tyrone: St John the Baptist
Muirhevnamore, Louth: Holy Family
Mullabrack, Armagh: St James'
Mullavilly (Kilmore) Armagh: Church of the
Immaculate Conception
Mullinahoe, Ardboe: Blessed Sacrament
Portadown William St: St Patrick's
Portadown: St John the Baptist
Tandragee, Armagh: St James'
The Loup, Derry: St Patrick's

Diocese of Cashel and Emly
Thurles Cathedral

Diocese of Cork & Ross

Ballincollig: Christ of our Light
Ballincollig: SS Mary & John
Ballydehob: St Brigid's
Ballyphehane: Church of the Assumption
Ballyvolane: St Oliver's
Blackrock Road: St Joseph's
Clonakily: Immaculate Conception
Cork City, Roman Street: SS Mary & Anne
Curraheen: The Real Presence
Douglas: St Columba's
Drimoleague: All Saints
Drinagh: Sacred Heart
Farren, Ovens; Immaculate Conception
Innishannon: St Mary's
Kinsale: St John the Baptist
Rochestown Road: St Patrick's
Sunday's Well: St Vincent's
Turners Cross: Christ the King

Diocese of Dublin
Arklow: SS Mary & Peter
Aughrim Street, Dublin: The Holy Family
Ballaly: Ascension of the Lord
Ballinteer: St John The Evangelist
Ballybrack: SS Alphonsus & Columba
Ballyfermot: Our Lady of the Assumption
Ballygall: Our Lady of Divine Grace
Ballyroan: Church of the Holy Spirit
Beaumont: The Navity of Our Lord
Blanchardstown: St Brigid's

Bluebell: Our Lady of the Wayside
Booterstown: Church of the Assumption
Brackenstown: St Cronin's
Bray: St Fergal's
Bray; Holy Redeemer
Bray: Our Lady of Peace
Cabra West: Most Precious Blood
Castleknock: Our Lady Mother of the Church
Churchtown: The Good Shepherd
Clondalkin: Immaculate Conception
Clonskeagh: Immaculate Virgin Mary
Clontarf: St Anthony's
Clontarf: St John The Baptist
Coolock: St Brendan's
Crumlin: St Agnes's
Dalkey: Assumption of the BVM
Dollymount: St Gabriel's
Dominick Street: St Saviour's
Drumcondra: Corpus Christi
Dundrum: Holy Cross
Dun Laoghaire: St Michael's
Edenmore: St Monica's
Enniskerry: St Mary's
Fairview: Church of the Visitation
Francis Street: St Nicholas of Myra
Gardiner Street: St Francis Xavier
Glasnevin: Our Lady of Dolours
Glendalough: St Kevin's
Grange Park: St Benedict's
Greystones: The Holy Rosary

Catholic churches with loop systems

Harrington Street: St Kevin's
Howth: Church of the Assumption
Huntstown: Sacred Heart of Jesus
Inchicore: Mary Immaculate
Iona Road: St Columba's
Killester: St Brigid's
Killinarden: The Sacred Heart
Kilmacud/Stillorgan: St Laurence
Kilquade: St Patrick
Kimmage Manor: Church of the Holy Spirit
Laurel Lodge: St Thomas the Apostle
Lucan: St Mary's
Malahide: St Sylvester's
Marino: St Vincent de Paul
Maynooth: St Mary's
Mount Argus: St Paul of the Cross
Mourne Road: Our Lady of Good Council
Navan Road: Our Lady Help of Christians
North William Street: St Agatha's
Palmerstown: St Philomena
Phibsboro: St Peter's
Rathgar: Church of the Three Patrons
Ringsend: St Patrick's
Saggart: Nativity BVM
Sandyford: St Mary's
Sandymount: St Mary's Star of the Sea
Swords: St Columcille
Templeogue: St Pius X
Whitefriar Street: Our Lady of Mount Carmel
Willington, Orwell Rd: St Jude the Apostle

Westland Row: St Andrew's

Diocese of Elphin
Boyle: St Joseph's
Sligo Cathedral: Immaculate Conception
Sligo: St Anne's

Diocese of Galway
Galway: Cathedral
Galway: St Francis
Galway: St Patrick's
Galway: University Church
Knocknacarra: Parish Church
Moycullen: Parish Church
Renmore: Parish Church
Salthill: Parish Church

Diocese of Kildare & Leighlin
Allen: Holy Trinity
Ballinabrana: St Fintan's
Leighlin Bridge: St Laserian's

Diocese of Ossory
Hugginstown: Parish Church
Kilkenny: St Mary's Cathedral
Kilkenny: St Johns's
Stoneyford: Parish Church

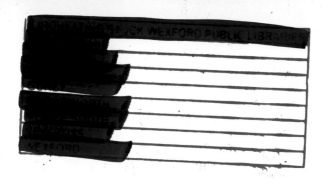